PLANT BASED RENAL DIET COOKBOOK FOR SENIORS

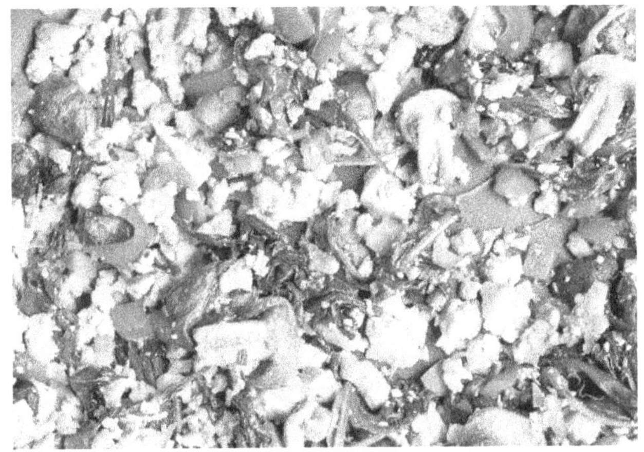

Discover Delicious and Easy to Make Kidney-friendly Vegan Recipes To Improve Your Kidney Health.

Joshua S. Gray

For more information or help feel free to contact me at:
joshuagrayhelpdesk@gmail.com

Table of Contents

INTRODUCTION

Ever wonder what actually nourishes and supports your body's complex needs as you age gracefully? Restrictions and sacrifice are widely regarded as the most effective ways to manage health conditions like renal disease. What if I told you that achieving better health doesn't have to involve deprivation?

As a professional dietitian, I've witnessed the common misconception that the best way to manage renal disease is to restrict your diet, leaving you craving flavors and variety. The truth is that a well-crafted plant-based renal diet can be more than just a solution; it can also be delicious and fulfilling.

Many seniors suffer from renal disease, a condition that makes dietary decisions extremely important. More than just a cookbook, this Plant-Based Renal Diet Cookbook for Seniors is a key to opening up a world of nourishing, plant-powered flavors that support your health objectives.

Imagine enjoying a plate full of colorful, nutrient-dense foods, with every bite a harmonious blend of flavors that have been chosen to support your kidneys and general health. What if I told you that this cookbook contains all the information you need to address your dietary worries and that it is specifically designed to provide seniors with renal disease with a plant-based diet?

You are about to go on a culinary adventure that aims to both celebrate and alleviate the challenges associated with renal disease. Feel the relief of finding a complete solution designed to transform your kitchen into a center for happiness and health.

Allow this book to be your companion and guide as you explore a world of delicious plant-based foods that put your health first without sacrificing flavor. As you embrace the possibilities of this special and nourishing culinary adventure, feel the pains of limitation melt away. This cookbook holds the secret to not only managing renal disease but also thriving on plant-based, flavorful foods. Prepare to transform your diet so that you can transform your health!

BENEFITS OF FOLLOWING PLANT BASED RENAL DIET RECIPES FOR SENIORS

Following a Plant-Based Renal Diet offers a multitude of benefits for seniors managing kidney health. Here are six key advantages:

1. **Kidney Support:** Plant-based diets, rich in fruits, vegetables, whole grains, and legumes, are naturally low in sodium and phosphorus, supporting kidney function. These foods provide essential nutrients without overloading the kidneys, promoting optimal renal health.

2. **Reduced Inflammation:** Plant-based diets have anti-inflammatory properties, which can be particularly beneficial for seniors with Chronic Kidney Disease (CKD). Lowering

inflammation levels may help manage symptoms and slow the progression of kidney damage.

3. **Heart Health:** Plant-based diets are inherently heart-healthy. By focusing on plant foods, seniors can reduce the intake of saturated fats and cholesterol, lowering the risk of cardiovascular complications often associated with renal disease.

4. **Blood Pressure Management:** Hypertension is a common complication of CKD. Plant-based diets, known for their ability to lower blood pressure, can be an effective tool in managing this aspect of kidney health, reducing strain on the cardiovascular system.

5. **Weight Management:** Maintaining a healthy weight is crucial for individuals with renal disease. Plant-based diets, high in fiber

and low in calorie density, can support weight management, preventing obesity-related complications that can exacerbate kidney issues.

6. **Balanced Nutrition:** A well-structured Plant-Based Renal Diet ensures seniors receive a balanced intake of essential nutrients. This approach provides vitamins, minerals, and antioxidants vital for overall health, supporting not only the kidneys but also the entire body.

Adopting a Plant-Based Renal Diet for seniors is a proactive step towards enhancing overall well-being. Beyond its positive impact on kidney health, this dietary approach contributes to improved cardiovascular health, inflammation reduction, and weight management. Embracing plant-based recipes tailored for renal health is a flavorful and nourishing way for seniors to prioritize their long-term vitality.

SHOPPING LIST

Creating a shopping list for a Plant-Based Renal Diet involves selecting nutrient-dense, kidney-friendly foods. Here's a comprehensive list to get you started:

1. Fruits:

- Apples

- Berries (blueberries, strawberries)

- Cherries

- Pineapple

- Watermelon

2. Vegetables:

- Spinach

- Kale

- Bell peppers

- Cauliflower

- Zucchini

3. Whole Grains:

- Quinoa

- Brown rice

- Whole wheat pasta

- Barley

- Bulgur

4. Legumes:

- Chickpeas

- Lentils

- Black beans

- Kidney beans

- Pinto beans

5. Nuts and Seeds:

- Almonds

- Walnuts

- Chia seeds

- Flaxseeds

- Pumpkin seeds

6. Plant-Based Protein:

   - Tofu

   - Tempeh

   - Edamame

7. Healthy Oils:

   - Olive oil

   - Avocado oil

8. Dairy Alternatives:

   - Almond milk

   - Soy milk

9. Herbs and Spices:

   - Basil

   - Cilantro

   - Turmeric

   - Cumin

   - Garlic powder

10. Low-Sodium Condiments:

- Balsamic vinegar

- Mustard

- Salsa (low sodium)

- Low-sodium soy sauce

11. Plant-Based Snacks:

- Air-popped popcorn

- Rice cakes

- Hummus

- Veggie chips

12. Beverages:

- Herbal teas

- Green tea

- Water

13. Sweeteners:

- Agave nectar

- Maple syrup

14. Fresh Herbs:

- Parsley

- Mint

- Dill

15. Whole Wheat Bread:

- Whole grain or whole wheat bread

16. Cruciferous Vegetables:

- Broccoli

- Brussels sprouts

- Cabbage

17. Avocado:

- Avocados

18. Plant-Based Proteins (Frozen):

- Veggie burgers

- Plant-based meat substitutes

19. Canned Tomatoes:

- Diced tomatoes (low sodium)

20. Dark Chocolate (Moderation):

- Dark chocolate (70% cocoa or higher)

Remember to choose low-sodium options and consult with a healthcare professional or dietitian for personalized advice based on individual dietary needs. This shopping list provides a foundation for creating delicious and kidney-friendly plant-based meals for seniors.

BREAKFAST RECIPES

1. Oatmeal with Berries and Almonds

- ½ cup steel-cut oats

- 1 cup almond milk

- ½ cup mixed berries

- 1 tablespoon chopped almonds

1. Cook oats in almond milk until creamy.

2. Top with mixed berries and chopped almonds.

Nutritional Value:

- Calories: Approximately 300 kcal

- Protein: 10g

- Fiber: 8g

- Healthy Fats: 7g

- Calcium: 150mg

- Iron: 2mg

Cooking Time: 15 minutes

2.   Chia Seed Pudding

- 3 tablespoons chia seeds

- 1 cup coconut milk

- ½ teaspoon vanilla extract

- ¼ cup fresh mango chunks

1. Mix chia seeds, coconut milk, and vanilla. Refrigerate overnight.

2. Top with fresh mango before serving.

- Calories: Approximately 250 kcal

- Protein: 5g

- Fiber: 12g

- Healthy Fats: 15g

- Vitamin C: 30mg

- Calcium: 200mg

Prep Time: 5 minutes + Refrigeration

3. Vegan Tofu Scramble

- ½ cup firm tofu (crumbled)

- ¼ cup diced bell peppers

- ¼ cup spinach

- 1 teaspoon turmeric

- Salt and pepper to taste

1.   Sauté tofu, bell peppers, and spinach with turmeric, salt, and pepper until cooked.

- Calories: Approximately 180 kcal

- Protein: 15g

- Fiber: 4g

- Healthy Fats: 10g

- Iron: 3mg

- Vitamin A: 800 IU

Cooking Time: 10 minutes

4. Whole Grain Toast with Hummus and Tomato

Ingredients:

- 2 slices whole-grain bread

- 2 tablespoons hummus

- 1 medium tomato (sliced)

- Fresh basil leaves for garnish

Instructions:

1. Toast bread, spread hummus, and top with tomato slices.

2. Garnish with fresh basil.

Nutritional Value:

- Calories: Approximately 200 kcal

- Protein: 8g

- Fiber: 6g

- Healthy Fats: 5g

- Vitamin C: 15mg

- Iron: 1.5mg

Prep Time: 5 minutes

5.   Blueberry Banana Smoothie Bowl

- 1 frozen banana
- ½ cup blueberries
- ½ cup spinach
- ½ cup almond milk
- 2 tablespoons rolled oats

1. Blend banana, blueberries, spinach, almond milk, and rolled oats until smooth.
2. Pour into a bowl.

Nutritional Value:

- Calories: Approximately 220 kcal

- Protein: 6g

- Fiber: 8g

- Healthy Fats: 4g

- Vitamin C: 25mg

- Calcium: 150mg

Prep Time: 5 minutes

6. Brown Rice Porridge with Cinnamon

Ingredients:

- ½ cup brown rice (cooked)

- 1 cup soy milk

- ½ teaspoon cinnamon

- 1 tablespoon raisins

Instructions:

1. Combine cooked brown rice, soy milk, cinnamon, and raisins.

2. Heat until warm.

Nutritional Value:

- Calories: Approximately 250 kcal

- Protein: 8g

- Fiber: 5g

- Healthy Fats: 4g

- Calcium: 180mg

Iron: 2.5mg

Cooking Time: 10 minutes

7. Spinach and Mushroom Vegan Omelette

- ½ cup chickpea flour

- ½ cup water

- ¼ cup chopped spinach

- ¼ cup sliced mushrooms

- ¼ cup diced tomatoes

1. Whisk chickpea flour and water until smooth.

2. Pour onto a hot pan and add spinach, mushrooms, and tomatoes.

3. Cook until set, then fold.

Nutritional Value:

- Calories: Approximately 220 kcal

- Protein: 12g

- Fiber: 6g

- Healthy Fats: 5g

- Iron: 3mg

- Vitamin A: 1000 IU

Cooking Time: 15 minutes

8.   Coconut Yogurt Parfait

- 1 cup coconut yogurt

- ½ cup granola

- ½ cup mixed berries

- 1 tablespoon shredded coconut

1. Layer coconut yogurt, granola, mixed berries, and shredded coconut.

2. Repeat as desired.

- Calories: Approximately 280 kcal

- Protein: 5g

- Fiber: 7g

- Healthy Fats: 10g

- Calcium: 200mg

- Vitamin C: 20mg

Prep Time: 5 minutes

9. Cauliflower Breakfast Burrito

- 1 cup cauliflower rice

- ¼ cup black beans (canned, rinsed)

- ¼ cup salsa

- Whole-grain tortilla

1. Sauté cauliflower rice, black beans, and salsa.

2. Fill a tortilla and fold into a burrito.

- Calories: Approximately 240 kcal

- Protein: 10g

- Fiber: 8g

- Healthy Fats: 5g

- Vitamin C: 15mg

- Iron: 2.5mg

Cooking Time: 10 minutes

10. Peanut Butter Banana Toast

Ingredients:

- 2 slices whole-grain bread

- 2 tablespoons peanut butter

- 1 banana (sliced)

- Drizzle of honey (optional)

Instructions:

1. Toast bread, spread peanut butter, top with banana slices, and drizzle with honey if desired.

Nutritional Value:

- Calories: Approximately 320 kcal

- Protein: 9g

- Fiber: 7g

- Healthy Fats: 12g

- Potassium: 400mg

- Iron: 1.8mg

Prep Time: 5 minutes

LUNCH RECIPES

1.   Quinoa Salad with Roasted Vegetables

Ingredients:

- 1 cup quinoa

- 2 cups mixed veggies like zucchini, bell peppers, and cherry tomatoes

- 2 tablespoons olive oil

- 1 tablespoon balsamic vinegar

- Salt and pepper to taste

Instructions:

1. Cook quinoa according to package instructions.

2. Toss mixed vegetables with olive oil, roast until tender.

3. Mix quinoa, roasted vegetables, and balsamic vinegar. Season with salt and pepper.

Nutritional Value:

- Calories: Approximately 280 kcal

- Protein: 8g

- Fiber: 10g

- Healthy Fats: 10g

- Vitamin C: 40mg

- Iron: 3mg

Cooking Time: 30 minutes

2. Lentil and Vegetable Stew

Ingredients:

- 1 cup green lentils

- 2 cups vegetable broth

- 1 cup carrots (diced)

- 1 cup celery (chopped)

- 1 cup kale (chopped)

- 1 teaspoon cumin

- Salt and pepper to taste

Instructions:

1. Rinse lentils and cook with vegetable broth until tender.

2. Add carrots, celery, kale, cumin, salt, and pepper.

3. Simmer until vegetables are cooked.

Nutritional Value:

- Calories: Approximately 220 kcal

- Protein: 15g

- Fiber: 12g

- Healthy Fats: 2g

- Iron: 4mg

- Vitamin A: 5000 IU

Cooking Time: 40 minutes

3. Chickpea and Spinach Curry

- 1 cup chickpeas (canned, rinsed)

- 1 cup spinach

- 1 cup tomatoes (diced)

- ½ cup onion (chopped)

- 1 teaspoon curry powder

- 1 tablespoon coconut oil

Instructions:

1. Sauté onions in coconut oil until golden.

2. Add chickpeas, tomatoes, and curry powder. Cook until tomatoes break down.

3. Stir in spinach and cook until wilted.

Nutritional Value:

- Calories: Approximately 260 kcal

- Protein: 11g

- Fiber: 9g

- Healthy Fats: 7g

- Vitamin C: 25mg

- Iron: 3.5mg

Cooking Time: 20 minutes

4. Sweet Potato and Black Bean Wrap

Ingredients:

- 1 large sweet potato (cooked and mashed)

- 1 cup black beans (canned, rinsed)

- ½ cup corn kernels

- 2 whole-grain tortillas

- ¼ cup salsa

- Fresh cilantro for garnish

Instructions:

1. Mix mashed sweet potato, black beans, and corn.

2. Spread the mixture onto tortillas, top with salsa, and garnish with cilantro.

3. Roll into wraps.

Nutritional Value:

- Calories: Approximately 300 kcal

- Protein: 10g

- Fiber: 12g

- Healthy Fats: 5g

- Vitamin A: 8000 IU

- Iron: 2.5mg

Prep Time: 15 minutes

5. Mushroom and Spinach Quiche

Ingredients:

- 1 cup mushrooms (sliced)

- 2 cups spinach

- 1 cup chickpea flour

- 1 ½ cups almond milk

- ½ teaspoon garlic powder

- Salt and pepper to taste

Instructions:

1. Sauté mushrooms and spinach until wilted.

2. Whisk chickpea flour, almond milk, garlic powder, salt, and pepper.

3. Pour the mixture into a baking dish, add sautéed mushrooms and spinach. Bake until set.

Nutritional Value:

- Calories: Approximately 230 kcal

- Protein: 12g

- Fiber: 8g

- Healthy Fats: 6g

- Iron: 3mg

- Vitamin D: 100 IU

Cooking Time: 35 minutes

6. Cauliflower and Chickpea Salad

- 1 cup cauliflower florets (roasted)

- 1 cup chickpeas (canned, rinsed)

- ½ cup cucumber (diced)

- ¼ cup red onion (finely chopped)

- 2 tablespoons olive oil

- 1 tablespoon lemon juice

Instructions:

1. Roast cauliflower until golden.

2. Combine roasted cauliflower, chickpeas, cucumber, red onion, olive oil, and lemon juice.

- Calories: Approximately 240 kcal

- Protein: 9g

- Fiber: 10g

- Healthy Fats: 10g

- Vitamin C: 30mg

- Iron: 2.5mg

Cooking Time: 25 minutes

7. Veggie Burger with Avocado

Ingredients:

- 2 plant-based burger patties

- 2 whole-grain burger buns

- 1 avocado (sliced)

- 1 cup lettuce leaves

- Tomato slices and mustard for garnish

Instructions:

1. Cook burger patties according to package instructions.

2. Toast burger buns, assemble with burger patties, avocado slices, lettuce, tomato, and mustard.

Nutritional Value:

- Calories: Approximately 320 kcal

- Protein: 15g

- Fiber: 8g

- Healthy Fats: 10g

- Vitamin A: 1200 IU

- Iron: 4mg

Cooking Time: 15 minutes

8.   Pasta Primavera with Pesto

- 2 cups whole-grain pasta

- 1 cup mixed vegetables (broccoli, cherry tomatoes, bell peppers)

- 2 tablespoons pesto sauce

- 1 tablespoon olive oil

- Salt and pepper to taste

Instructions:

1. Cook pasta, adding mixed vegetables in the last 3 minutes.

2. Drain, toss with pesto sauce, olive oil, salt, and pepper.

Nutritional Value:

- Calories: Approximately 290 kcal

- Protein: 9g

- Fiber: 10g

- Healthy Fats: 8g

- Vitamin C: 35mg

- Iron: 2.5mg

Cooking Time: 15 minutes

9. Tofu Stir-Fry with Brown Rice

Ingredients:

- 1 cup tofu (cubed)

- 1 cup broccoli florets

- ½ cup snap peas

- ¼ cup soy sauce

- 1 tablespoon sesame oil

- 1 tablespoon ginger (minced)

Instructions:

1. Sauté tofu until golden. Add broccoli, snap peas, soy sauce, sesame oil, and ginger. Stir-fry until vegetables are tender.

- Calories: Approximately 260 kcal

- Protein: 15g

- Fiber: 6g

- Healthy Fats: 10g

- Iron: 3mg

- Calcium: 200mg

Cooking Time: 20 minutes

10. Stuffed Bell Peppers with Quinoa and Black Beans

Ingredients:

- 2 bell peppers (halved)

- 1 cup cooked quinoa

- ½ cup black beans (canned, rinsed)

- ½ cup corn kernels

- ¼ cup salsa

- ¼ teaspoon cumin

Instructions:

1. Preheat oven to 375°F (190°C).

2. Mix cooked quinoa, black beans, corn, salsa, and cumin.

3. Stuff bell peppers with the quinoa mixture. Bake until peppers are tender.

Nutritional Value:

- Calories: Approximately 290 kcal

- Protein: 11g

- Fiber: 12g

- Healthy Fats: 4g

- Vitamin C: 80mg

- Iron: 2.5mg

Cooking Time: 30 minutes

DINNER RECIPES

1. Miso-Glazed Eggplant with Quinoa

Ingredients:

- 2 medium-sized eggplants (sliced)

- ¼ cup miso paste

- 2 tablespoons maple syrup

- 1 cup quinoa

- 2 cups vegetable broth

- Sesame seeds for garnish

Instructions:

1. Mix miso paste and maple syrup to make the glaze.

2. Brush eggplant slices with the miso glaze and bake until tender.

3. Cook quinoa in vegetable broth. Serve the eggplant over quinoa and garnish with sesame seeds.

Nutritional Value:

- Calories: Approximately 320 kcal

- Protein: 10g

- Fiber: 8g

- Healthy Fats: 6g

- Magnesium: 120mg

- Iron: 3mg

Cooking Time: 35 minutes

2. Cilantro-Lime Chickpea Salad

- 2 cups chickpeas (canned, rinsed)

- 1 cup cucumber (diced)

- 1 cup cherry tomatoes (halved)

- ¼ cup red onion (finely chopped)

- ¼ cup fresh cilantro (chopped)

- 2 tablespoons olive oil

- Juice of 1 lime

Instructions:

1. Combine chickpeas, cucumber, tomatoes, red onion, and cilantro.

2. Drizzle with olive oil and lime juice. Toss gently.

Nutritional Value:

- Calories: Approximately 280 kcal

- Protein: 12g

- Fiber: 10g

- Healthy Fats: 7g

- Vitamin C: 30mg

- Iron: 2.5mg

Prep Time: 15 minutes

3. Spaghetti Squash with Tomato Basil Sauce

Ingredients:

- 1 medium-sized spaghetti squash

- 2 cups tomatoes (diced)

- ¼ cup fresh basil (chopped)

- 2 cloves garlic (minced)

- 1 tablespoon olive oil

- Salt and pepper to taste

Instructions:

1. Roast spaghetti squash until tender and scrape out the strands.

2. Sauté tomatoes, basil, and garlic in olive oil. Season with salt and pepper.

3. Serve the tomato basil sauce over spaghetti squash.

Nutritional Value:

- Calories: Approximately 250 kcal

- Protein: 5g

- Fiber: 8g

- Healthy Fats: 6g

- Vitamin A: 2000 IU

- Iron: 2mg

Cooking Time: 40 minutes

4. Stuffed Portobello Mushrooms

Ingredients:

- 4 large portobello mushrooms

- 1 cup quinoa (cooked)

- ½ cup black beans (canned, rinsed)

- ½ cup corn kernels

- ¼ cup diced tomatoes

- ¼ teaspoon cumin

- 1 tablespoon balsamic vinegar

Instructions:

1. Preheat the oven to 375°F (190°C).

2. Remove stems from mushrooms, brush with balsamic vinegar, and bake until tender.

3. Mix quinoa, black beans, corn, tomatoes, and cumin. Stuff mushrooms with the mixture.

Nutritional Value:

- Calories: Approximately 300 kcal

- Protein: 12g

- Fiber: 10g

- Healthy Fats: 5g

- Vitamin C: 20mg

- Iron: 2.5mg

Cooking Time: 25 minutes

5.   Lemon Herb Baked Tofu

- 1 block firm tofu (pressed and cubed)

- 2 tablespoons lemon juice

- 1 tablespoon olive oil

- 1 teaspoon dried thyme

- 1 teaspoon dried rosemary

- Salt and pepper to taste

1. Preheat the oven to 375°F (190°C).

2. Toss tofu cubes with lemon juice, olive oil, thyme, rosemary, salt, and pepper.

3. Bake until tofu is golden and slightly crispy.

Nutritional Value:

- Calories: Approximately 230 kcal

- Protein: 15g

- Fiber: 5g

- Healthy Fats: 10g

- Calcium: 300mg

- Iron: 2mg

Cooking Time: 30 minutes

6. Broccoli and Red Lentil Soup

Ingredients:

- 1 cup red lentils

- 4 cups vegetable broth

- 2 cups broccoli florets

- ½ cup carrots (diced)

- ½ cup celery (chopped)

- 1 teaspoon turmeric

- Salt and pepper to taste

Instructions:

1. Rinse lentils and cook in vegetable broth until soft.

2. Add broccoli, carrots, celery, turmeric, salt, and pepper. Simmer until vegetables are tender.

Nutritional Value:

- Calories: Approximately 240 kcal

- Protein: 15g

- Fiber: 10g

- Healthy Fats: 2g

- Iron: 4mg

- Vitamin C: 40mg

Cooking Time: 35 minutes

7. Zucchini Noodles with Pesto

Ingredients:

- 2 medium-sized zucchinis (spiralized)

- ¼ cup pine nuts

- 1 cup fresh basil

- 2 cloves garlic

- ¼ cup nutritional yeast

- ¼ cup olive oil

Instructions:

1. Spiralize zucchinis into noodles.

2. Blend pine nuts, basil, garlic, nutritional yeast, and olive oil to make pesto.

3. Toss zucchini noodles with pesto.

- Calories: Approximately 260 kcal

- Protein: 8g

- Fiber: 6g

- Healthy Fats: 20g

- Iron: 2mg

- Calcium: 80mg

Prep Time: 20 minutes

8.   Tomato and Chickpea Stew

Ingredients:

- 2 cups tomatoes (diced)

- 1 cup chickpeas (canned, rinsed)

- ½ cup onion (chopped)

- ½ cup bell peppers (sliced)

- 1 tablespoon tomato paste

- 1 teaspoon Italian seasoning

- Salt and pepper to taste

Instructions:

1. Sauté onions and bell peppers until softened.

2. Add tomatoes, chickpeas, tomato paste, Italian seasoning, salt, and pepper. Simmer until flavors meld.

Nutritional Value:

- Calories: Approximately 220 kcal

- Protein: 10g

- Fiber: 8g

- Healthy Fats: 3g

- Vitamin C: 25mg

- Iron: 2mg

Cooking Time: 25 minutes

9. Stir-Fried Bok Choy with Tofu

- 1 cup tofu (cubed)

- 2 cups bok choy (chopped)

- ½ cup shiitake mushrooms (sliced)

- 1 tablespoon soy sauce

- 1 tablespoon sesame oil

- 1 tablespoon ginger (minced)

1.   Sauté tofu until golden. Add bok choy, mushrooms, soy sauce, sesame oil, and ginger. Stir-fry until vegetables are tender.

Nutritional Value:

- Calories: Approximately 230 kcal

- Protein: 12g

- Fiber: 6g

- Healthy Fats: 10g

- Iron: 2.5mg

- Calcium: 200mg

Cooking Time: 20 minutes

10. Moroccan-Inspired Couscous Bowl

Ingredients:

- 1 cup whole wheat couscous

- 1 cup chickpeas (canned, rinsed)

- ½ cup dried apricots (chopped)

- ¼ cup almonds (sliced)

- 1 teaspoon cumin

- 1 teaspoon cinnamon

- 1 tablespoon olive oil

Instructions:

1. Cook couscous according to package instructions.

2. Mix cooked couscous, chickpeas, dried apricots, almonds, cumin, cinnamon, and olive oil.

Nutritional Value:

- Calories: Approximately 290 kcal

- Protein: 10g

- Fiber: 8g

- Healthy Fats: 6g

- Iron: 2.5mg

- Vitamin A: 1000 IU

Cooking Time: 15 minutes

SNACK RECIPES

1. Roasted Chickpeas with Herbs

Ingredients:

- 1 cup chickpeas (canned, rinsed)

- 1 tablespoon olive oil

- 1 teaspoon dried rosemary

- 1 teaspoon dried thyme

- Salt and pepper to taste

Instructions:

1. Preheat the oven to 400°F (200°C).

2. Toss chickpeas with olive oil, rosemary, thyme, salt, and pepper.

3. Roast until chickpeas are crispy.

Nutritional Value:

- Calories: Approximately 150 kcal

- Protein: 7g

- Fiber: 5g

- Healthy Fats: 6g

- Iron: 2mg

- Magnesium: 60mg

Cooking Time: 30 minutes

2. Baked Sweet Potato Fries

- 2 medium-sized sweet potatoes (cut into fries)

- 1 tablespoon olive oil

- ½ teaspoon paprika

- ½ teaspoon garlic powder

- Salt and pepper to taste

Instructions:

1. Preheat the oven to 425°F (220°C).

2. Toss sweet potato fries with olive oil, paprika, garlic powder, salt, and pepper.

3. Bake until fries are golden and crispy.

Nutritional Value:

- Calories: Approximately 120 kcal

- Protein: 2g

- Fiber: 4g

- Healthy Fats: 4g

- Vitamin A: 16000 IU

- Potassium: 250mg

Cooking Time: 25 minutes

3. Cucumber and Hummus Bites

Ingredients:

- 1 medium-sized cucumber (sliced)

- ¼ cup hummus

- Cherry tomatoes for garnish

- Fresh parsley for garnish

Instructions:

1. Slice cucumber into rounds.

2. Top each cucumber slice with a small spoonful of hummus.

3. Garnish with cherry tomatoes and fresh parsley.

Nutritional Value:

- Calories: Approximately 80 kcal

- Protein: 3g

- Fiber: 2g

- Healthy Fats: 4g

- Vitamin C: 15mg

- Calcium: 30mg

Prep Time: 10 minutes

4.   Almond and Berry Trail Mix

Ingredients:

- ½ cup almonds

- ¼ cup dried blueberries

- ¼ cup dried cranberries

- ¼ cup pumpkin seeds

Instructions:

1. Mix almonds, dried blueberries, dried cranberries, and pumpkin seeds.
2. Portion into snack-sized servings.

Nutritional Value:

- Calories: Approximately 200 kcal

- Protein: 7g

- Fiber: 5g

- Healthy Fats: 12g

- Iron: 1.5mg

- Magnesium: 90mg

Prep Time: 5 minutes

5. Apple Slices with Almond Butter

- 1 medium-sized apple (sliced)

- 2 tablespoons almond butter

- Cinnamon for sprinkling

Instructions:

1. Slice apple into wedges.

2. Spread almond butter on apple slices.

3. Sprinkle with cinnamon.

Nutritional Value:

- Calories: Approximately 180 kcal

- Protein: 3g

- Fiber: 5g

- Healthy Fats: 10g

- Vitamin C: 8mg

- Potassium: 200mg

Prep Time: 5 minutes

6.   Chia Seed Pudding Parfait

Ingredients:

- 3 tablespoons chia seeds

- 1 cup almond milk

- ½ teaspoon vanilla extract

- ¼ cup fresh berries

- 2 tablespoons granola

Instructions:

1. Mix chia seeds, almond milk, and vanilla. Refrigerate until set.

2. Layer chia pudding with fresh berries and granola.

Nutritional Value:

- Calories: Approximately 220 kcal

- Protein: 5g

- Fiber: 10g

- Healthy Fats: 7g

- Calcium: 150mg

- Iron: 2mg

Prep Time: 5 minutes + Refrigeration

7.   Greek Salad Skewers

- Cherry tomatoes

- Cucumber chunks

- Kalamata olives

- Vegan feta cheese cubes

- Fresh oregano for garnish

1. Thread cherry tomatoes, cucumber chunks, olives, and feta cheese cubes onto skewers.

2. Garnish with fresh oregano.

- Calories: Approximately 160 kcal

- Protein: 4g

- Fiber: 3g

- Healthy Fats: 10g

- Vitamin C: 20mg

- Calcium: 100mg

Prep Time: 15 minutes

8. Rice Cake with Avocado and Tomato

- 1 rice cake

- ½ avocado (sliced)

- ½ cup cherry tomatoes (halved)

- Sprinkle of sea salt and black pepper

1. Spread avocado slices on the rice cake.

2. Top with cherry tomato halves.

3. Sprinkle with sea salt and black pepper.

- Calories: Approximately 140 kcal

- Protein: 3g

- Fiber: 5g

- Healthy Fats: 7g

- Vitamin C: 10mg

- Potassium: 250mg

Prep Time: 5 minutes

9. Carrot Sticks with Hummus

Ingredients:

- 1 cup carrot sticks

- ¼ cup hummus

- Fresh parsley for garnish

Instructions:

1. Arrange carrot sticks on a plate.

2. Serve with a side of hummus.

3. Garnish with fresh parsley.

Nutritional Value:

- Calories: Approximately 90 kcal

- Protein: 3g

- Fiber: 4g

- Healthy Fats: 5g

- Vitamin A: 16000 IU

- Calcium: 40mg

Prep Time: 5 minutes

10. Mango Salsa with Baked Pita Chips

Ingredients:

- 1 ripe mango (diced)

- ¼ cup red onion (finely chopped)

- ¼ cup cilantro (chopped)

- 1 tablespoon lime juice

- Whole-grain pita bread (cut into chips)

Instructions:

1. Mix mango, red onion, cilantro, and lime juice to make salsa.

2. Bake whole-grain pita bread until crispy.

3. Serve mango salsa with baked pita chips.

Nutritional Value:

- Calories: Approximately 160 kcal

- Protein: 3g

- Fiber: 4g

- Healthy Fats: 2g

- Vitamin C: 45mg

- Potassium: 200mg

Prep Time: 10 minutes + Baking

DESSERT RECIPES

1.   Chia Seed and Berry Parfait

Ingredients:

- 3 tablespoons chia seeds

- 1 cup almond milk

- ½ teaspoon vanilla extract

- ½ cup mixed berries

- 1 tablespoon chopped nuts for garnish

Instructions:

1. Mix chia seeds, almond milk, and vanilla. Refrigerate until set.

2. Layer chia pudding with mixed berries.

3. Garnish with chopped nuts.

Nutritional Value:

- Calories: Approximately 180 kcal

- Protein: 5g

- Fiber: 10g

- Healthy Fats: 7g

- Calcium: 150mg

- Iron: 2mg

Prep Time: 5 minutes + Refrigeration

2.   Baked Apple with Cinnamon

Ingredients:

- 1 medium-sized apple

- ½ teaspoon cinnamon

- 1 tablespoon chopped walnuts

- 1 teaspoon maple syrup

Instructions:

1. Core the apple and sprinkle with cinnamon.

2. Bake until tender.

3. Top with chopped walnuts and drizzle with maple syrup.

Nutritional Value:

- Calories: Approximately 120 kcal

- Protein: 1g

- Fiber: 4g

- Healthy Fats: 5g

- Vitamin C: 8mg

- Potassium: 150mg

Cooking Time: 25 minutes

3.   Coconut Rice Pudding

Ingredients:

- ½ cup Arborio rice

- 2 cups coconut milk

- ¼ cup maple syrup

- ½ teaspoon vanilla extract

- ¼ cup shredded coconut for garnish

Instructions:

1. Cook Arborio rice in coconut milk until creamy.

2. Stir in maple syrup and vanilla extract.

3. Garnish with shredded coconut.

- Calories: Approximately 220 kcal

- Protein: 3g

- Fiber: 2g

- Healthy Fats: 10g

- Calcium: 20mg

- Iron: 1mg

Cooking Time: 30 minutes

4.   Banana-Oat Cookies

Ingredients:

- 2 ripe bananas (mashed)

- 1 cup rolled oats

- ¼ cup chopped dates

- ¼ cup chopped walnuts

- ½ teaspoon cinnamon

Instructions:

1. Mix mashed bananas, rolled oats, dates, walnuts, and cinnamon.

2. Drop spoonfuls onto a baking sheet.

3. Bake until golden.

- Calories: Approximately 160 kcal

- Protein: 3g

- Fiber: 4g

- Healthy Fats: 5g

- Iron: 1.5mg

- Potassium: 200mg

Cooking Time: 15 minutes

5. Avocado Chocolate Mousse

Ingredients:

- 2 ripe avocados

- ¼ cup cocoa powder

- ¼ cup maple syrup

- ½ teaspoon vanilla extract

- Fresh berries for garnish

Instructions:

1. Blend avocados, cocoa powder, maple syrup, and vanilla until smooth.

2. Chill in the refrigerator.

3. Garnish with fresh berries before serving.

- Calories: Approximately 180 kcal

- Protein: 3g

- Fiber: 7g

- Healthy Fats: 10g

- Iron: 1.5mg

- Potassium: 400mg

Prep Time: 10 minutes + Chilling

6.   Pumpkin Chia Pudding

Ingredients:

- 3 tablespoons chia seeds

- 1 cup almond milk

- ¼ cup canned pumpkin puree

- ½ teaspoon pumpkin spice

- 1 tablespoon chopped pecans for garnish

Instructions:

1. Mix chia seeds, almond milk, pumpkin puree, and pumpkin spice. Refrigerate until set.

2. Sprinkle with chopped pecans before serving.

- Calories: Approximately 200 kcal

- Protein: 5g

- Fiber: 8g

- Healthy Fats: 8g

- Calcium: 150mg

- Iron: 2mg

Prep Time: 5 minutes + Refrigeration

7.   Blueberry Oat Squares

- 1 cup rolled oats

- ½ cup whole wheat flour

- ¼ cup maple syrup

- ¼ cup applesauce

- ½ cup fresh blueberries

Instructions:

1. Mix rolled oats, whole wheat flour, maple syrup, and applesauce.

2. Fold in fresh blueberries.

3. Press into a baking dish and bake until firm.

- Calories: Approximately 180 kcal

- Protein: 4g

- Fiber: 5g

- Healthy Fats: 2g

- Iron: 1.5mg

- Potassium: 100mg

Cooking Time: 20 minutes

8.   Mango Sorbet

- 2 cups frozen mango chunks

- ¼ cup coconut water

- 1 tablespoon lime juice

- Fresh mint for garnish

Instructions:

1. Blend frozen mango chunks, coconut water, and lime juice until smooth.

2. Scoop into bowls and garnish with fresh mint.

Nutritional Value:

- Calories: Approximately 120 kcal

- Protein: 1g

- Fiber: 3g

- Healthy Fats: 1g

- Vitamin C: 45mg

- Potassium: 200mg

Prep Time: 5 minutes

9. Date and Walnut Energy Balls

Ingredients:

- 1 cup dates (pitted)

- ½ cup walnuts

- ¼ cup shredded coconut

- ½ teaspoon vanilla extract

- Pinch of sea salt

Instructions:

1. Blend dates, walnuts, shredded coconut, vanilla extract, and sea salt until a dough forms.

2. Roll into bite-sized balls.

Nutritional Value:

- Calories: Approximately 160 kcal

- Protein: 3g

- Fiber: 4g

- Healthy Fats: 8g

- Iron: 1.5mg

- Potassium: 200mg

Prep Time: 10 minutes

10. Peach and Almond Crisp

Ingredients:

- 2 cups sliced peaches

- ¼ cup almond flour

- ¼ cup rolled oats

- 1 tablespoon maple syrup

- ½ teaspoon cinnamon

Instructions:

1. Mix sliced peaches, almond flour, rolled oats, maple syrup, and cinnamon.

2. Bake until the topping is golden and peaches are bubbly.

Nutritional Value:

- Calories: Approximately 140 kcal

- Protein: 3g

- Fiber: 4g

- Healthy Fats: 5g

- Vitamin C: 10mg

- Potassium: 180mg

Cooking Time: 30 minutes

30 Day Meal Plan

Week 1

Day 1

Breakfast: Oatmeal with Berries and Almonds

Lunch: Quinoa Salad with Roasted Vegetables

Dinner: Miso-Glazed Eggplant with Quinoa

Snack: Roasted Chickpeas with Herbs

Dessert: Chia Seed and Berry Parfait

Day 2

Breakfast: Chia Seed Pudding

Lunch: Lentil and Vegetable Stew

Dinner: Cilantro-Lime Chickpea Salad

Snack: Baked Sweet Potato Fries

Dessert: Baked Apple with Cinnamon

Day 3

Breakfast: Vegan Tofu Scramble

Lunch: Chickpea and Spinach Curry

Dinner: Spaghetti Squash with Tomato Basil Sauce

Snack: Cucumber and Hummus Bites

Dessert: Coconut Rice Pudding

Day 4

Breakfast: Whole Grain Toast with Hummus and Tomato

Lunch: Sweet Potato and Black Bean Wrap

Dinner: Stuffed Portobello Mushrooms

Snack: Almond and Berry Trail Mix

Dessert: Banana-Oat Cookies

Day 5

Breakfast: Blueberry Banana Smoothie Bowl

Lunch: Mushroom and Spinach Quiche

Dinner: Lemon Herb Baked Tofu

Snack: Apple Slices with Almond Butter

Dessert: Avocado Chocolate Mousse

Day 6

Breakfast: Brown Rice Porridge with Cinnamon

Lunch: Cauliflower and Chickpea Salad

Dinner: Broccoli and Red Lentil Soup

Snack: Chia Seed Pudding Parfait

Dessert: Pumpkin Chia Pudding

Day 7

Breakfast: Spinach and Mushroom Vegan Omelette

Lunch: Veggie Burger with Avocado

Dinner: Zucchini Noodles with Pesto

Snack: Greek Salad Skewers

Dessert: Blueberry Oat Squares

Week 2

Day 8

Breakfast: Coconut Yogurt Parfait

Lunch: Pasta Primavera with Pesto

Dinner: Tomato and Chickpea Stew

Snack: Rice Cake with Avocado and Tomato

Dessert: Mango Sorbet

Day 9

Breakfast: Cauliflower Breakfast Burrito

Lunch: Tofu Stir-Fry with Brown Rice

Dinner: Stir-Fried Bok Choy with Tofu

Snack: Carrot Sticks with Hummus

Dessert: Date and Walnut Energy Balls

Day 10

Breakfast: Peanut Butter Banana Toast

Lunch: Stuffed Bell Peppers with Quinoa and Black Beans

Dinner: Moroccan-Inspired Couscous Bowl

Snack: Mango Salsa with Baked Pita Chips

Dessert: Peach and Almond Crisp

Day 11

Breakfast: Blueberry Banana Smoothie Bowl

Lunch: Mushroom and Spinach Quiche

Dinner: Lemon Herb Baked Tofu

Snack: Apple Slices with Almond Butter

Dessert: Avocado Chocolate Mousse

Day 12

Breakfast: Brown Rice Porridge with Cinnamon

Lunch: Cauliflower and Chickpea Salad

Dinner: Broccoli and Red Lentil Soup

Snack: Chia Seed Pudding Parfait

Dessert: Pumpkin Chia Pudding

Breakfast: Spinach and Mushroom Vegan Omelette

Lunch: Veggie Burger with Avocado

Dinner: Zucchini Noodles with Pesto

Snack: Greek Salad Skewers

Dessert: Blueberry Oat Squares

Breakfast: Coconut Yogurt Parfait

Lunch: Pasta Primavera with Pesto

Dinner: Tomato and Chickpea Stew

Snack: Rice Cake with Avocado and Tomato

Dessert: Mango Sorbet

Week 3

Day 15

Breakfast: Cauliflower Breakfast Burrito

Lunch: Tofu Stir-Fry with Brown Rice

Dinner: Stir-Fried Bok Choy with Tofu

Snack: Carrot Sticks with Hummus

Dessert: Date and Walnut Energy Balls

Day 16

Breakfast: Peanut Butter Banana Toast

Lunch: Stuffed Bell Peppers with Quinoa and Black Beans

Dinner: Moroccan-Inspired Couscous Bowl

Snack: Mango Salsa with Baked Pita Chips

Dessert: Peach and Almond Crisp

Day 17

Breakfast: Oatmeal with Berries and Almonds

Lunch: Quinoa Salad with Roasted Vegetables

Dinner: Miso-Glazed Eggplant with Quinoa

Snack: Roasted Chickpeas with Herbs

Dessert: Chia Seed and Berry Parfait

Day 18

Breakfast: Chia Seed Pudding

Lunch: Lentil and Vegetable Stew

Dinner: Cilantro-Lime Chickpea Salad

Snack: Baked Sweet Potato Fries

Dessert: Baked Apple with Cinnamon

Day 19

Breakfast: Vegan Tofu Scramble

Lunch: Chickpea and Spinach Curry

Dinner: Spaghetti Squash with Tomato Basil Sauce

Snack: Cucumber and Hummus Bites

Dessert: Coconut Rice Pudding

Day 20

Breakfast: Whole Grain Toast with Hummus and Tomato

Lunch: Sweet Potato and Black Bean Wrap

Dinner: Stuffed Portobello Mushrooms

Snack: Almond and Berry Trail Mix

Dessert: Banana-Oat Cookies

Day 21

Breakfast: Blueberry Banana Smoothie Bowl

Lunch: Mushroom and Spinach Quiche

Dinner: Lemon Herb Baked Tofu

Snack: Apple Slices with Almond Butter

Dessert: Avocado Chocolate Mousse

Week 4

Day 22

Breakfast: Spinach and Mushroom Vegan Omelette

Lunch: Veggie Burger with Avocado

Dinner: Zucchini Noodles with Pesto

Snack: Greek Salad Skewers

Dessert: Blueberry Oat Squares

Day 23

Breakfast: Coconut Yogurt Parfait

Lunch: Pasta Primavera with Pesto

Dinner: Tomato and Chickpea Stew

Snack: Rice Cake with Avocado and Tomato

Dessert: Mango Sorbet

Day 24

Breakfast: Oatmeal with Berries and Almonds

Lunch: Quinoa Salad with Roasted Vegetables

Dinner: Miso-Glazed Eggplant with Quinoa

Snack: Roasted Chickpeas with Herbs

Dessert: Chia Seed and Berry Parfait

Day 25

Breakfast: Chia Seed Pudding

Lunch: Lentil and Vegetable Stew

Dinner: Cilantro-Lime Chickpea Salad

Snack: Baked Sweet Potato Fries

Dessert: Baked Apple with Cinnamon

Day 26

Breakfast: Whole Grain Toast with Hummus and Tomato

Lunch: Sweet Potato and Black Bean Wrap

Dinner: Stuffed Portobello Mushrooms

Snack: Almond and Berry Trail Mix

Dessert: Banana-Oat Cookies

Day 27

Breakfast: Blueberry Banana Smoothie Bowl

Lunch: Mushroom and Spinach Quiche

Dinner: Lemon Herb Baked Tofu

Snack: Apple Slices with Almond Butter

Dessert: Avocado Chocolate Mousse

Day 28

Breakfast: Cauliflower Breakfast Burrito

Lunch: Tofu Stir-Fry with Brown Rice

Dinner: Stir-Fried Bok Choy with Tofu

Snack: Carrot Sticks with Hummus

Dessert: Date and Walnut Energy Balls

Day 29

Breakfast: Peanut Butter Banana Toast

Lunch: Stuffed Bell Peppers with Quinoa and Black Beans

Dinner: Moroccan-Inspired Couscous Bowl

Snack: Mango Salsa with Baked Pita Chips

Dessert: Peach and Almond Crisp

Breakfast: Brown Rice Porridge with Cinnamon

Lunch: Cauliflower and Chickpea Salad

Dinner: Broccoli and Red Lentil Soup

Snack: Chia Seed Pudding Parfait

Dessert: Pumpkin Chia Pudding

CONCLUSION

I would like to thank you, dear reader, for starting this journey toward better renal health and for reading this entire Plant-Based Renal Diet Cookbook for Seniors. You are demonstrating a proactive approach to managing renal health in your golden years by adopting a plant-based lifestyle, which tells volumes about your commitment to well-being.

It is my sincere hope that the flavors of healthful, kidney-friendly ingredients bring you happiness and fulfillment as you explore the many and nourishing recipes found within these pages. I hope this cookbook proves to be a useful tool for you in your pursuit of a healthier way of living, helping you to make the shift to a plant-based renal diet both easy and enjoyable.

As a comprehensive solution to the difficulties that may arise from renal health concerns, I see this cookbook as more than just a compilation of recipes. Enable your body, mind, and soul to be nourished by the colorful selection of plant-based dishes, cultivating a sense of well-being that goes beyond restrictive eating.

Don't forget that every meal is a step toward better health. I therefore urge you to jump enthusiastically into this plant-based journey, armed with your newly acquired knowledge and some delicious recipes. Cheers to your well-being, energy, and the pleasure you derive from each delicious, kidney-friendly bite. I hope this cookbook holds the key to a brighter future and a restored sense of well-being.

My Little Request

Dear Reader,

Thanks for your purchase, hope you enjoyed reading.

Could you please take a few seconds to leave a positive feedback on this book?

It'll help reach more people and we can collectively help reverse this deadly disease.

Thank you.

BONUS: MEAL PLANNER JOURNAL

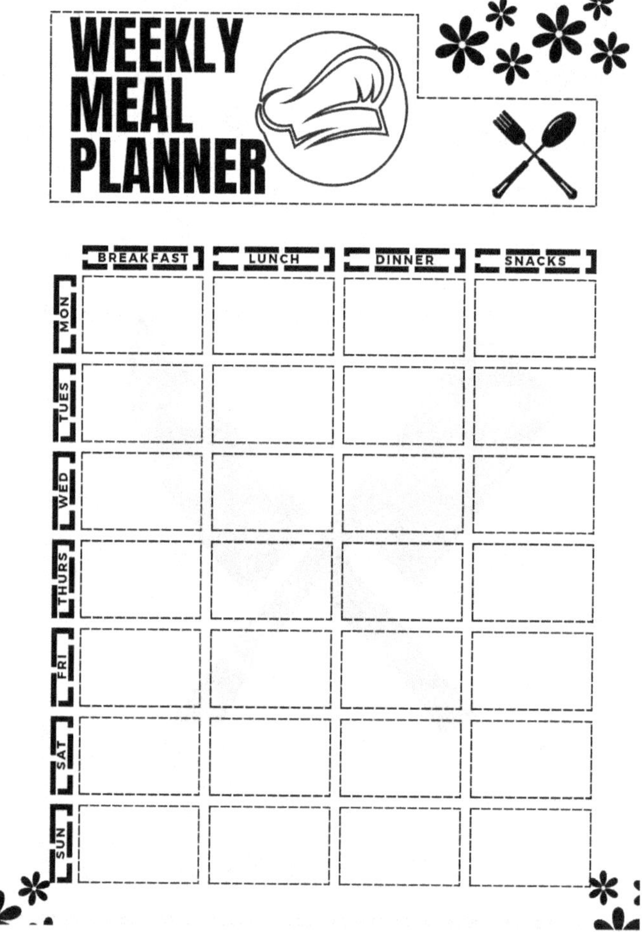

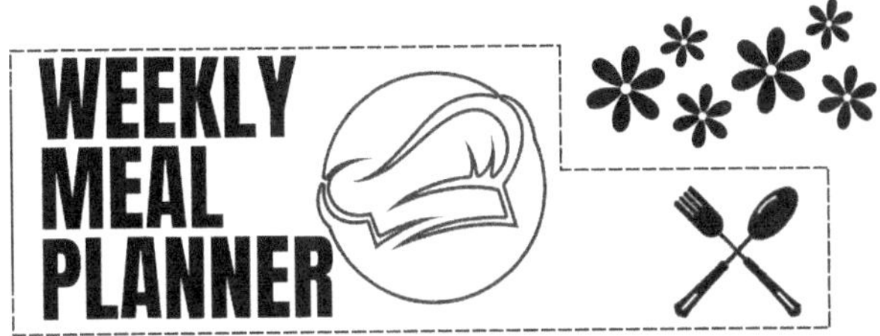

WEEKLY
MEAL
PLANNER

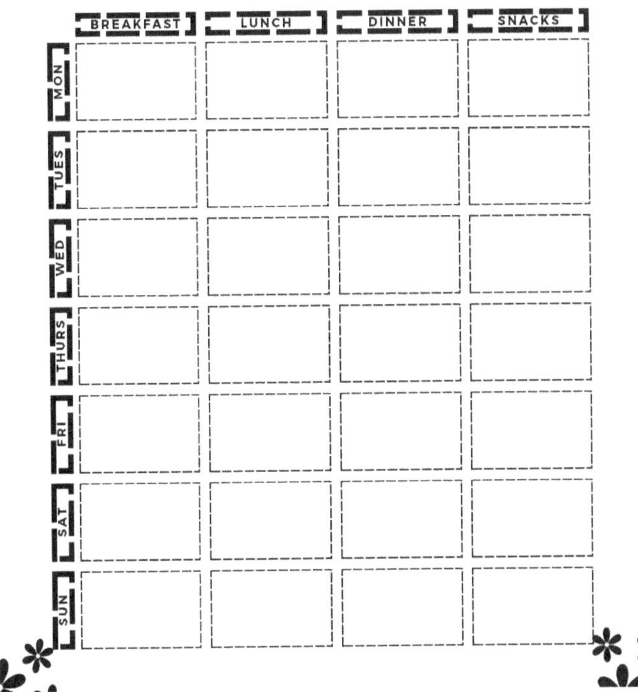

BREAKFAST
LUNCH
DINNER
SNACKS
MON
TUES
WED
THURS
FRI
SAT
SUN

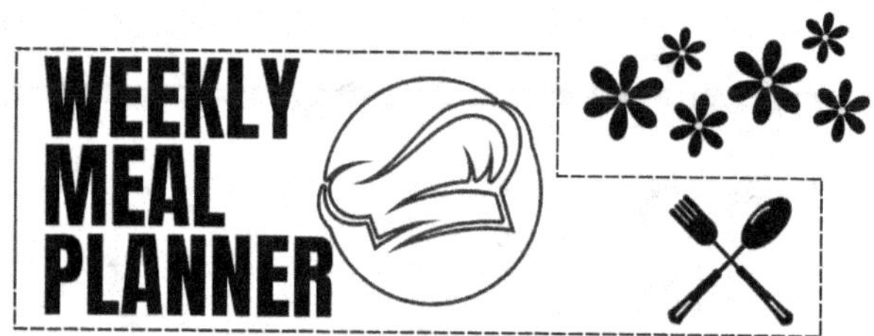

WEEKLY
MEAL
PLANNER

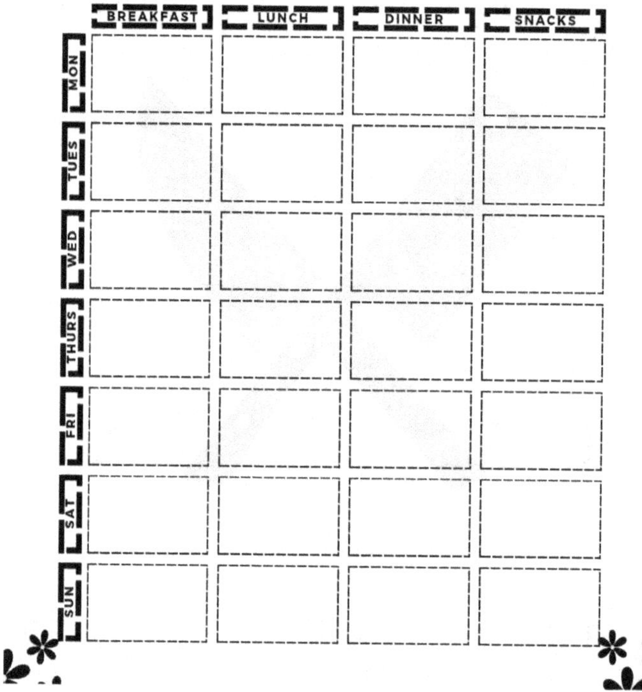

BREAKFAST
LUNCH
DINNER
SNACKS
MON
TUES
WED
THURS
FRI
SAT
SUN

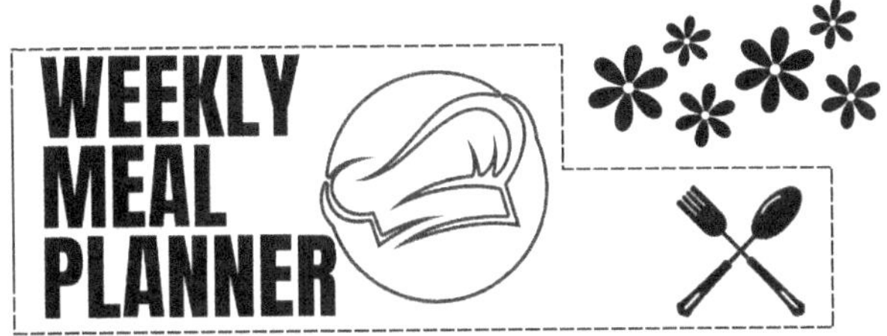
WEEKLY
MEAL
PLANNER

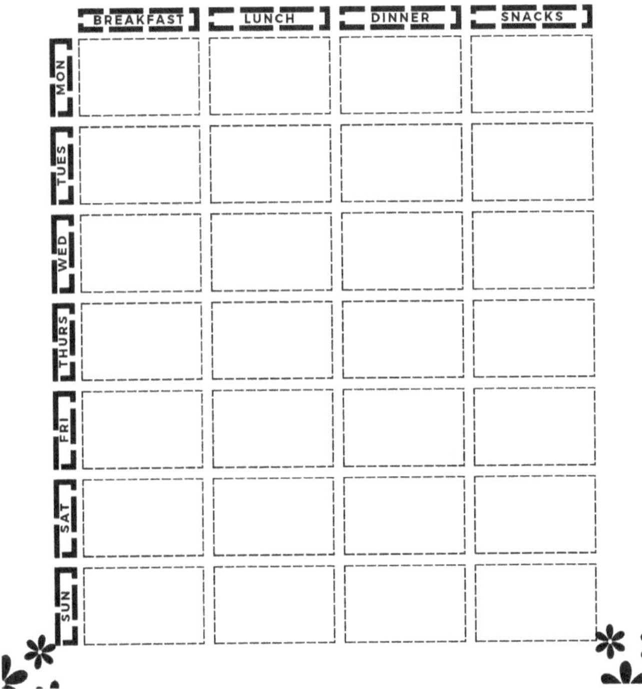
BREAKFAST
LUNCH
DINNER
SNACKS
MON
TUES
WED
THURS
FRI
SAT
SUN

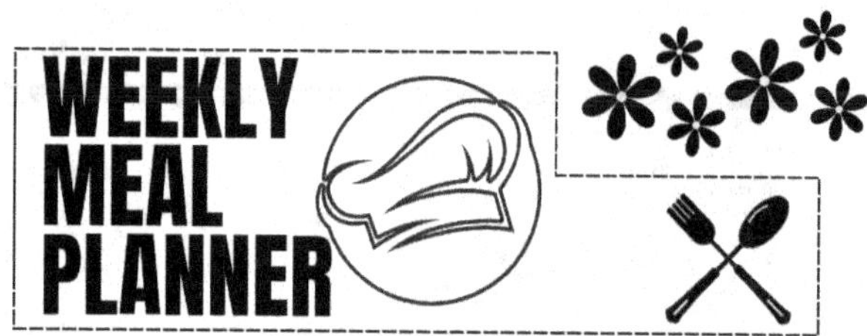

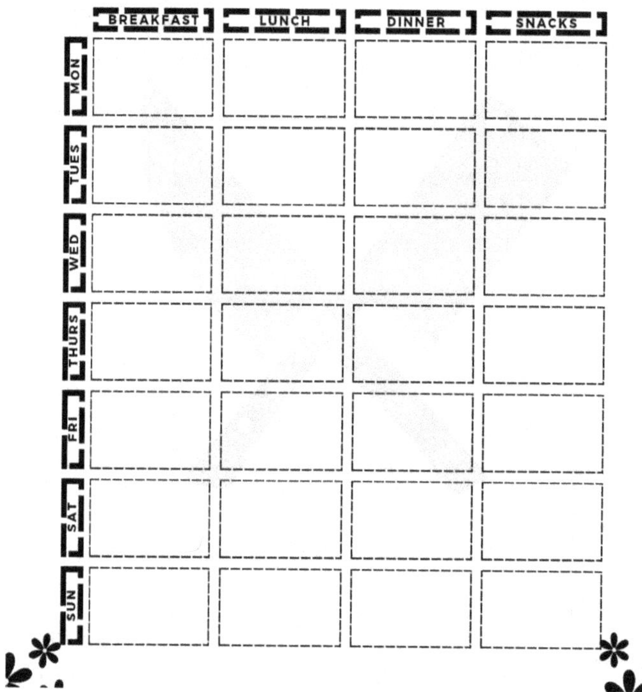

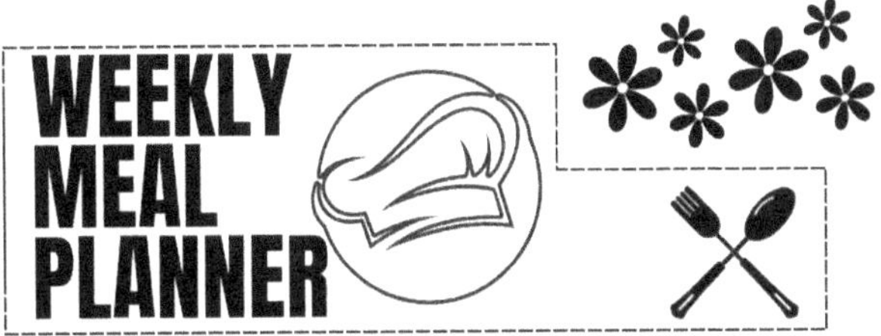

WEEKLY
MEAL
PLANNER

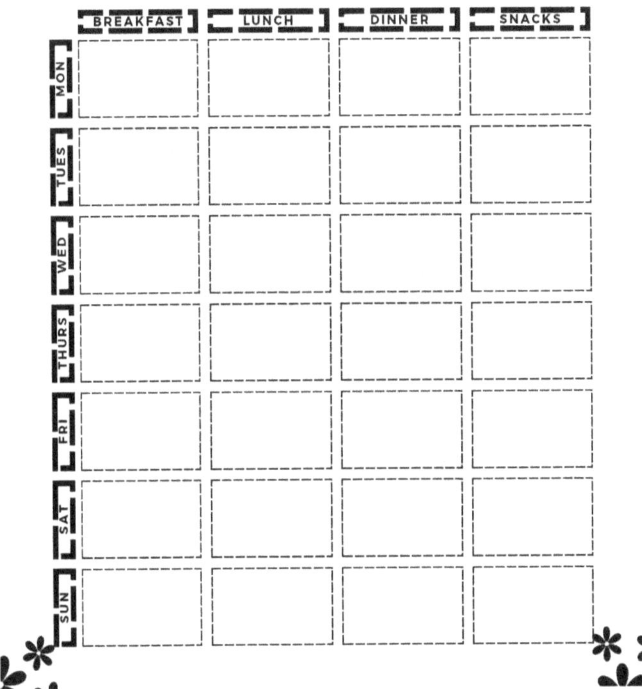

BREAKFAST
LUNCH
DINNER
SNACKS
MON
TUES
WED
THURS
FRI
SAT
SUN

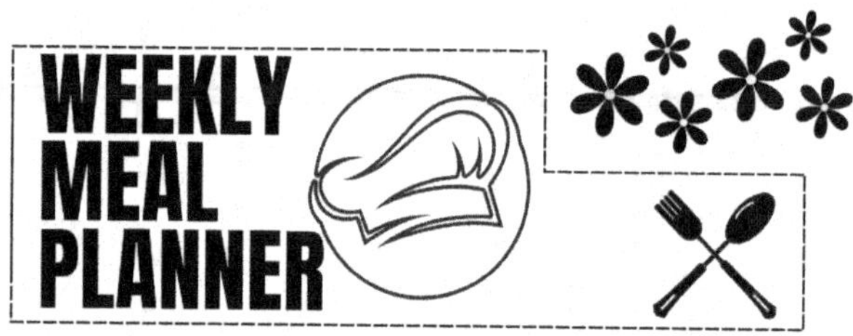

WEEKLY
MEAL
PLANNER

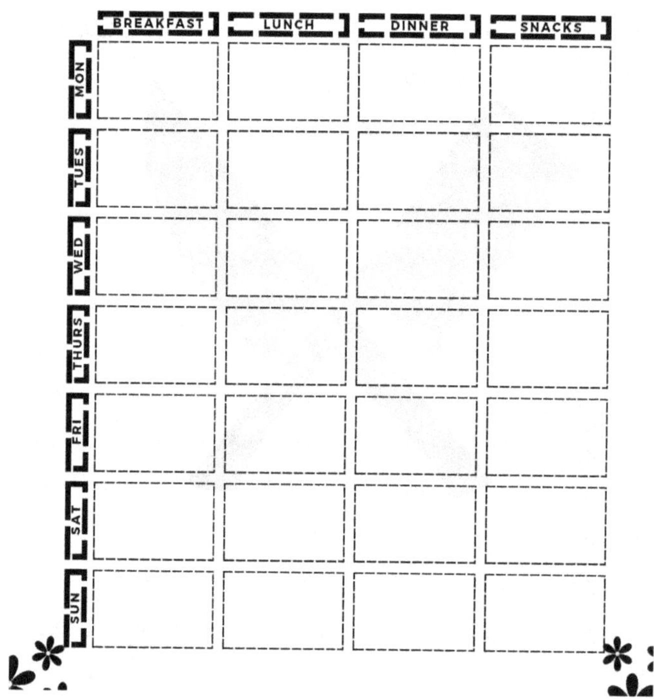

BREAKFAST
LUNCH
DINNER
SNACKS
MON
TUES
WED
THURS
FRI
SAT
SUN

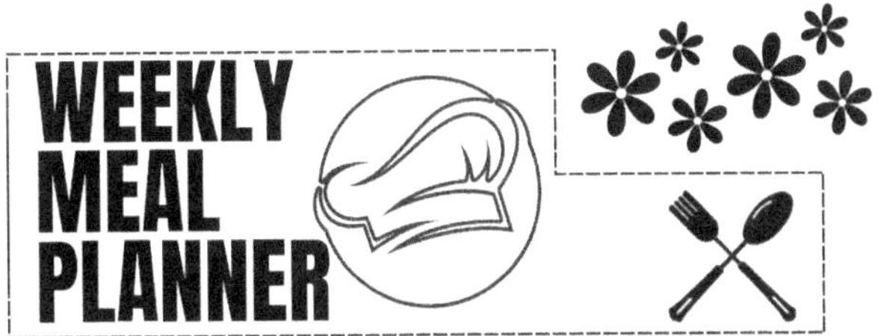
WEEKLY
MEAL
PLANNER

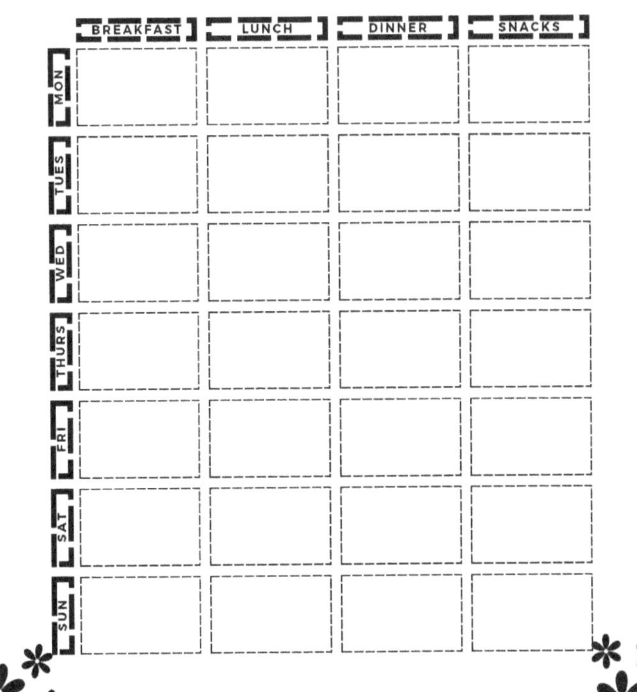
BREAKFAST
LUNCH
DINNER
SNACKS
MON
TUES
WED
THURS
FRI
SAT
SUN

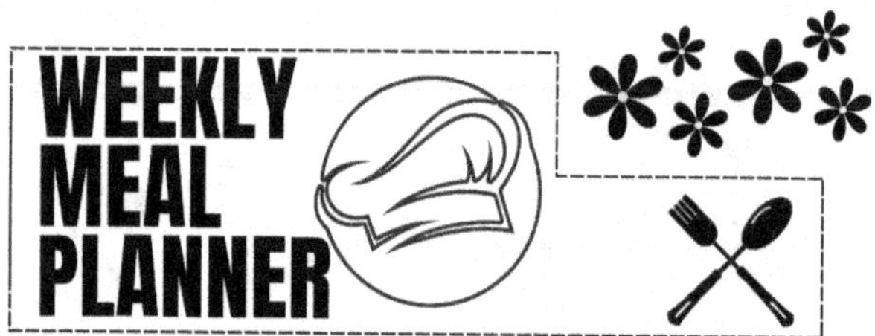

WEEKLY
MEAL
PLANNER

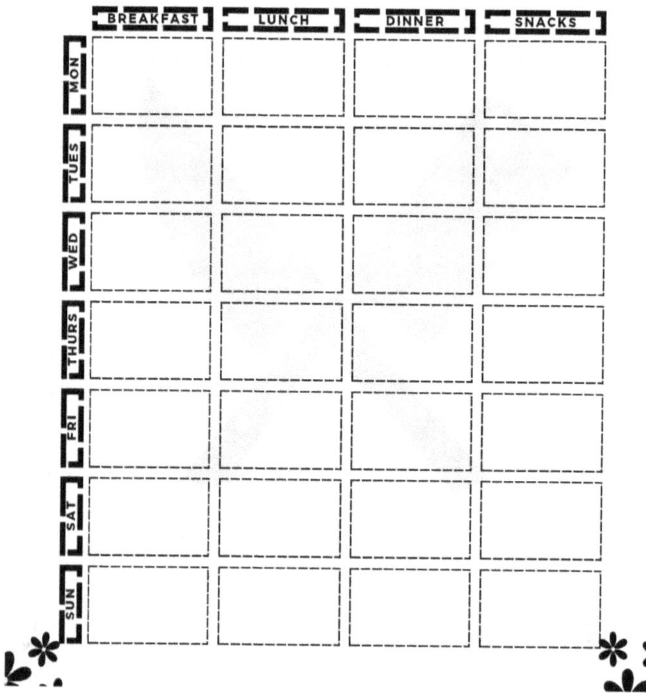

BREAKFAST
LUNCH
DINNER
SNACKS
MON
TUES
WED
THURS
FRI
SAT
SUN

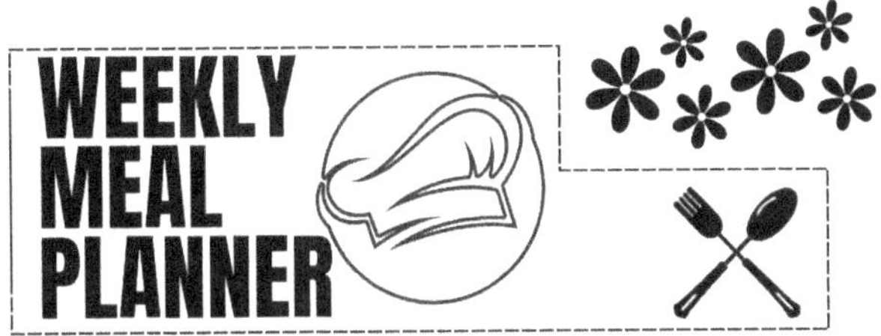

WEEKLY
MEAL
PLANNER

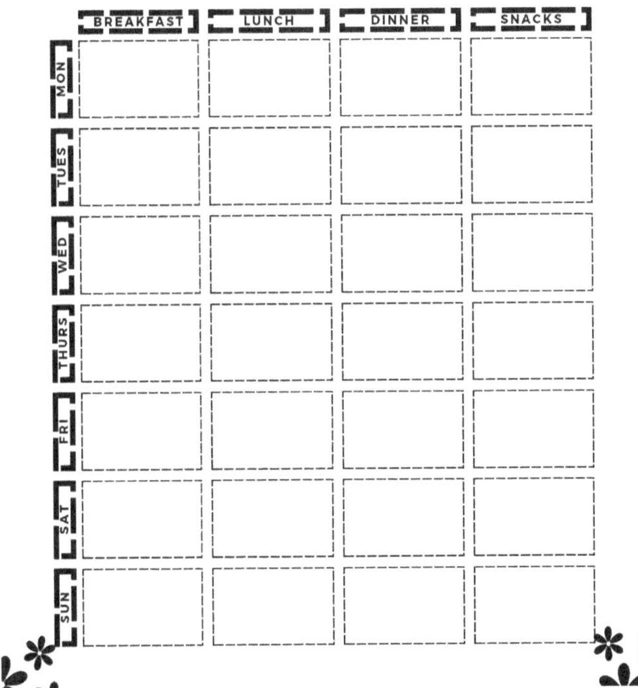

BREAKFAST
LUNCH
DINNER
SNACKS
MON
TUES
WED
THURS
FRI
SAT
SUN

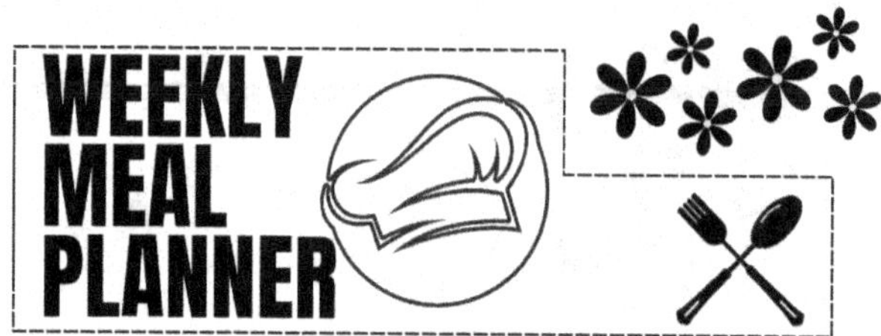

WEEKLY
MEAL
PLANNER

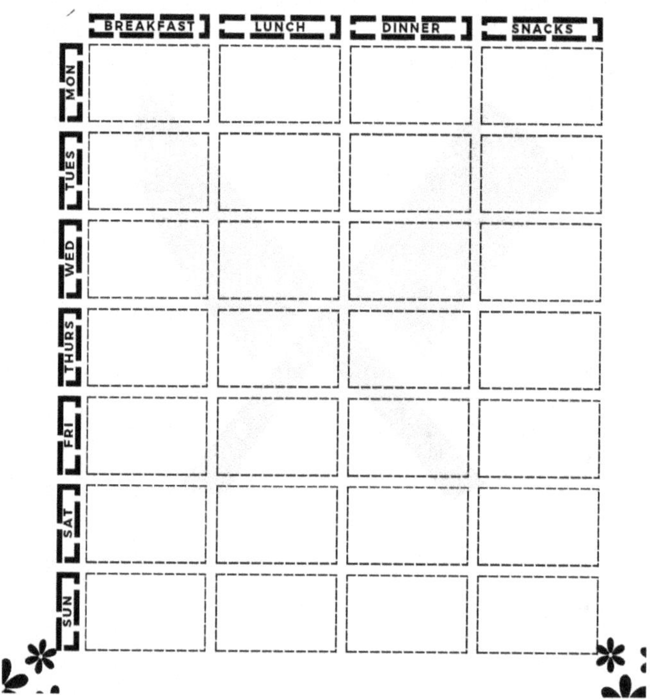

BREAKFAST
LUNCH
DINNER
SNACKS
MON
TUES
WED
THURS
FRI
SAT
SUN

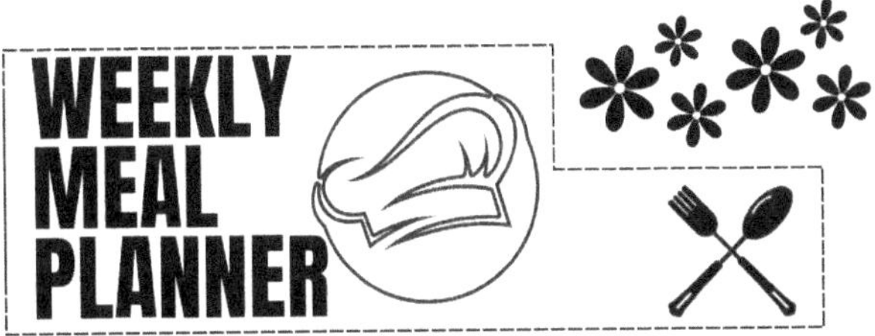

WEEKLY
MEAL
PLANNER

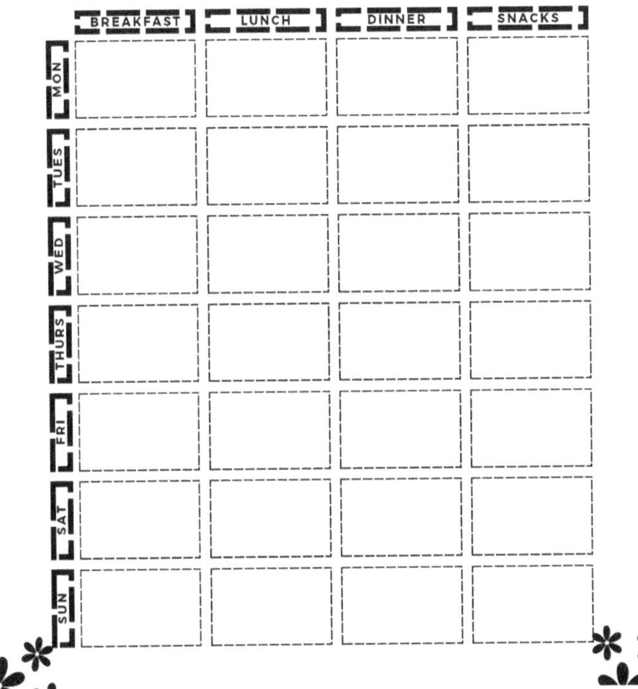

BREAKFAST
LUNCH
DINNER
SNACKS
MON
TUES
WED
THURS
FRI
SAT
SUN

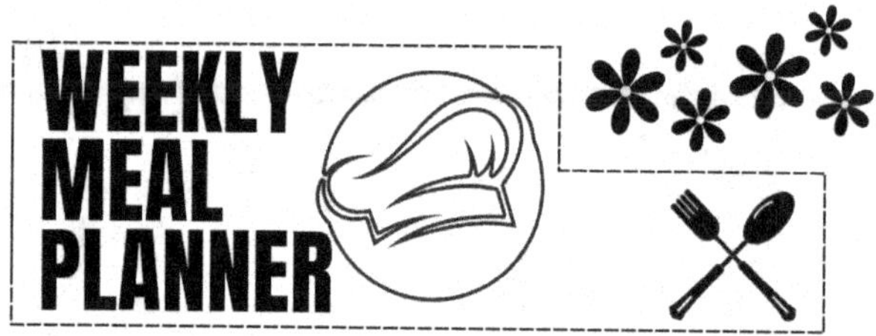
WEEKLY
MEAL
PLANNER

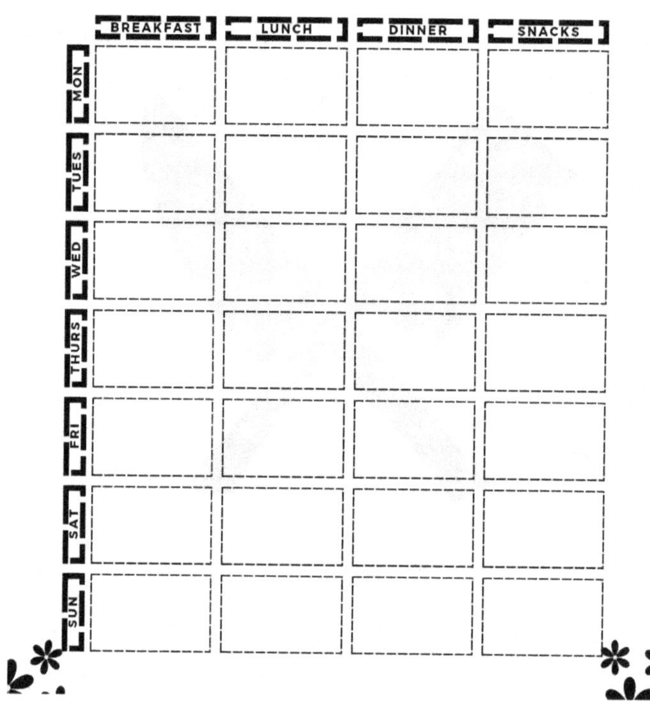
BREAKFAST
LUNCH
DINNER
SNACKS
MON
TUES
WED
THURS
FRI
SAT
SUN

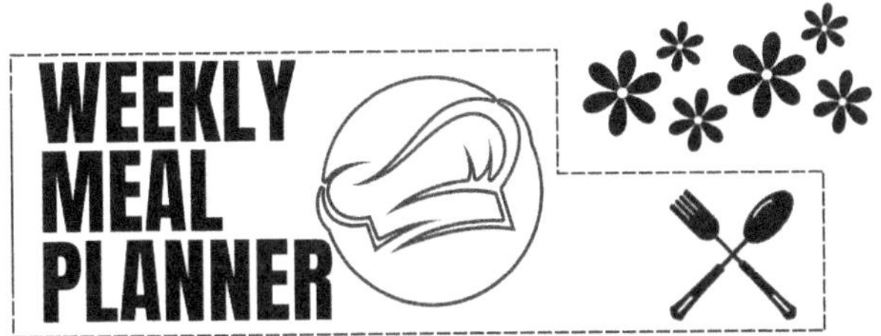

WEEKLY MEAL PLANNER

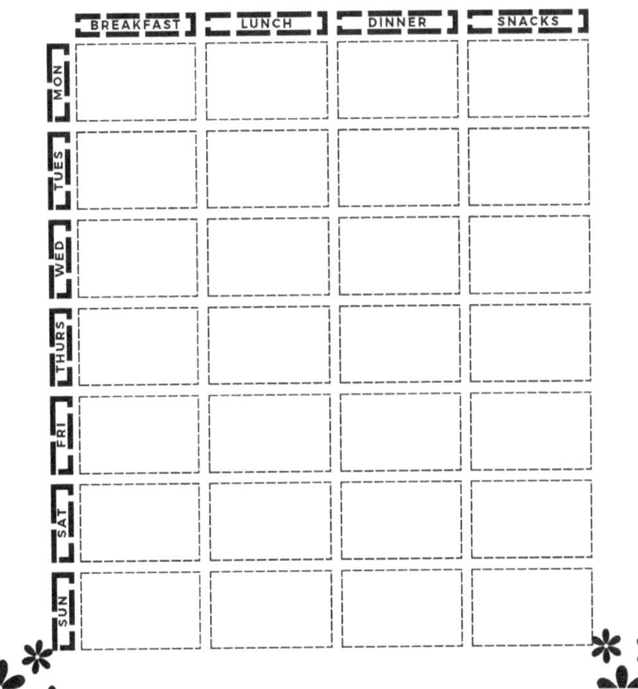

BREAKFAST
LUNCH
DINNER
SNACKS
MON
TUES
WED
THURS
FRI
SAT
SUN

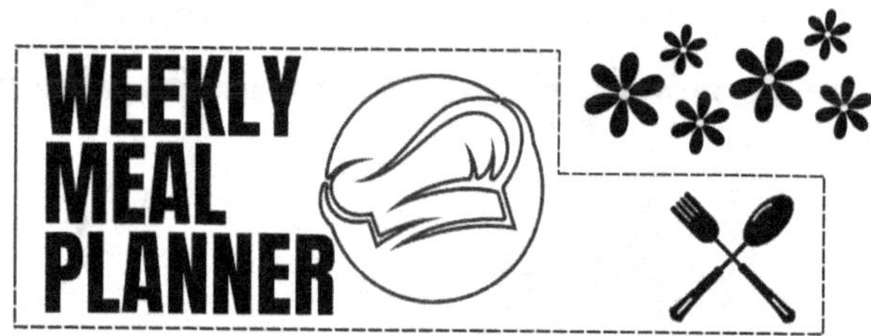

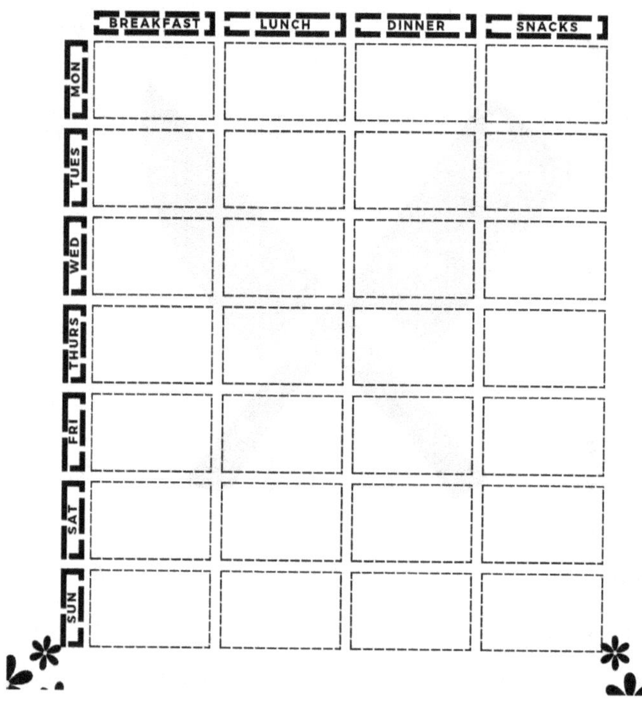
BREAKFAST
LUNCH
DINNER
SNACKS
MON
TUES
WED
THURS
FRI
SAT
SUN

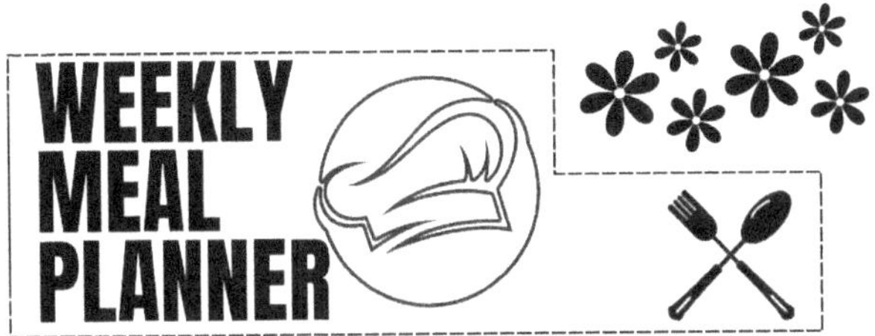

WEEKLY
MEAL
PLANNER

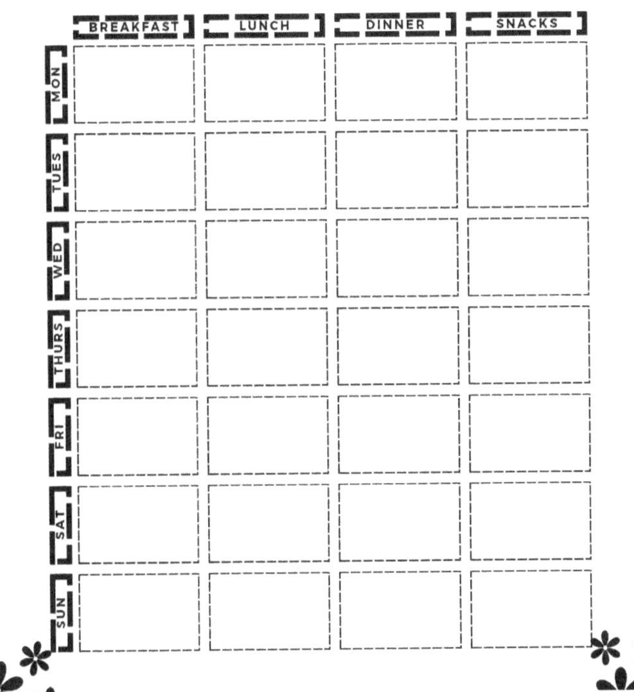

BREAKFAST
LUNCH
DINNER
SNACKS
MON
TUES
WED
THURS
FRI
SAT
SUN

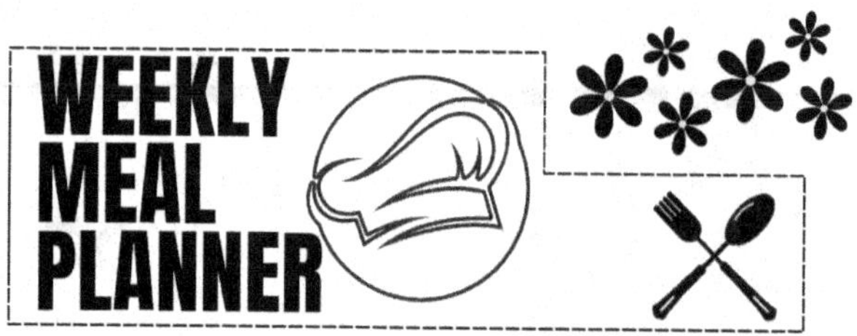

WEEKLY
MEAL
PLANNER

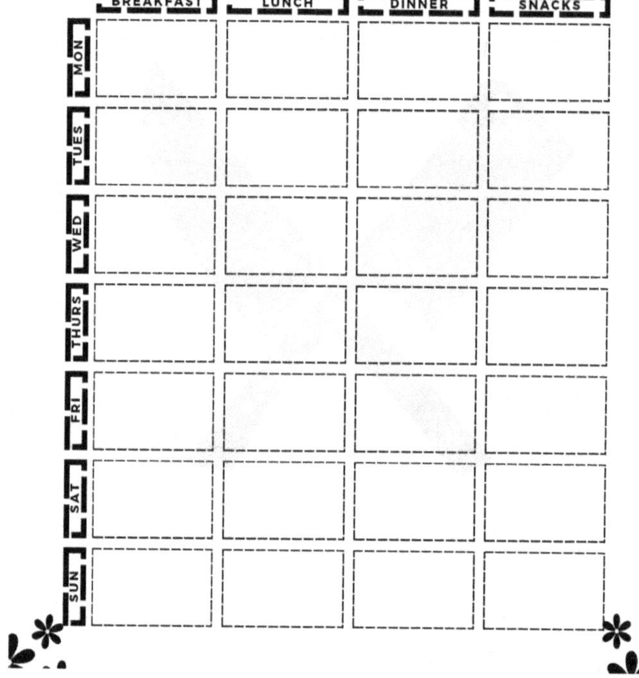

BREAKFAST
LUNCH
DINNER
SNACKS
MON
TUES
WED
THURS
FRI
SAT
SUN

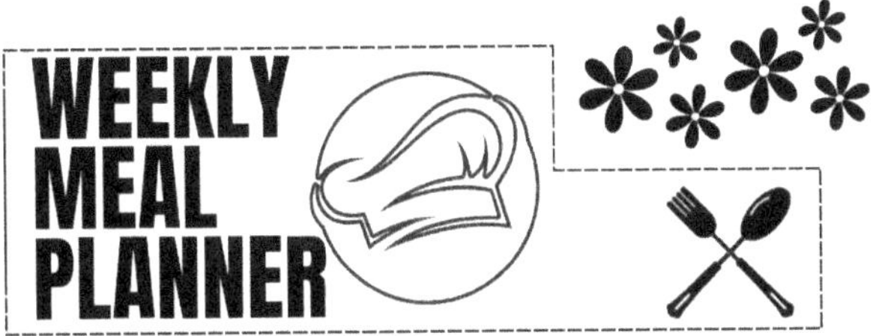

WEEKLY
MEAL
PLANNER

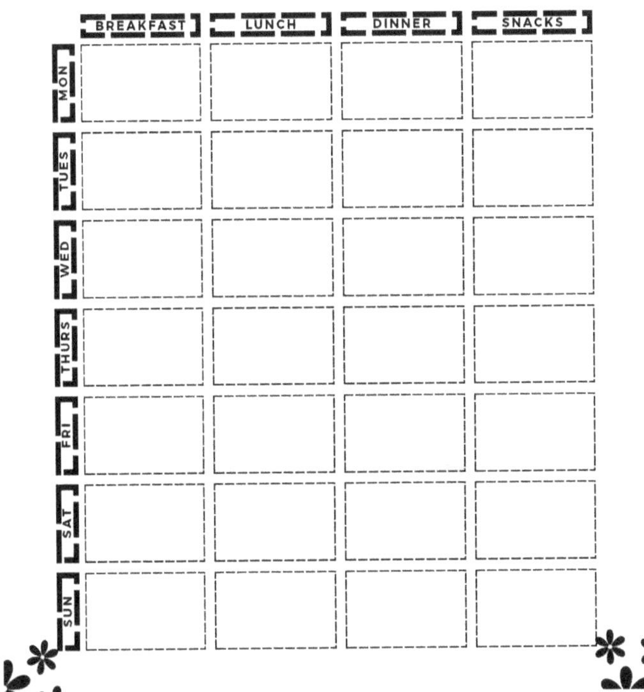

BREAKFAST
LUNCH
DINNER
SNACKS
MON
TUES
WED
THURS
FRI
SAT
SUN

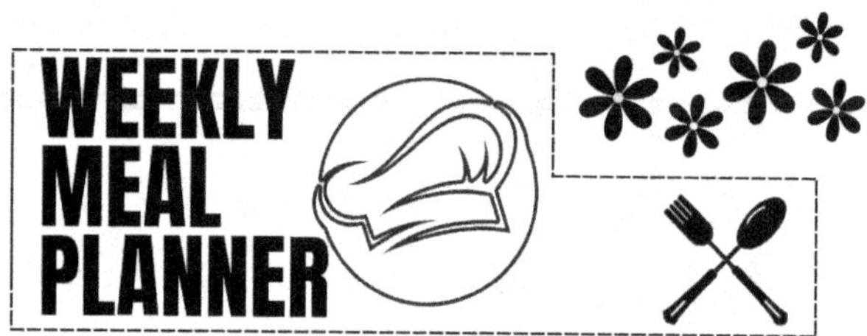

WEEKLY
MEAL
PLANNER

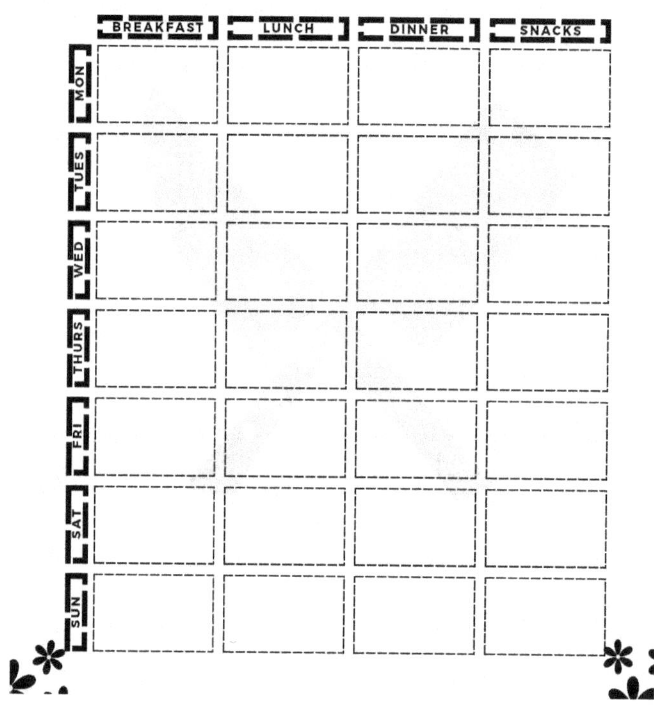

BREAKFAST
LUNCH
DINNER
SNACKS
MON
TUES
WED
THURS
FRI
SAT
SUN

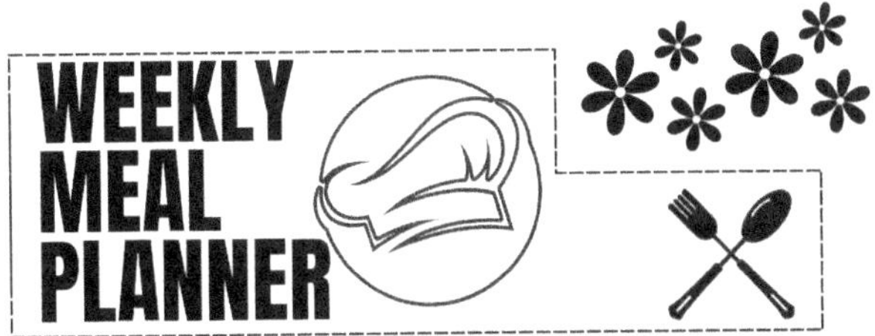

WEEKLY
MEAL
PLANNER

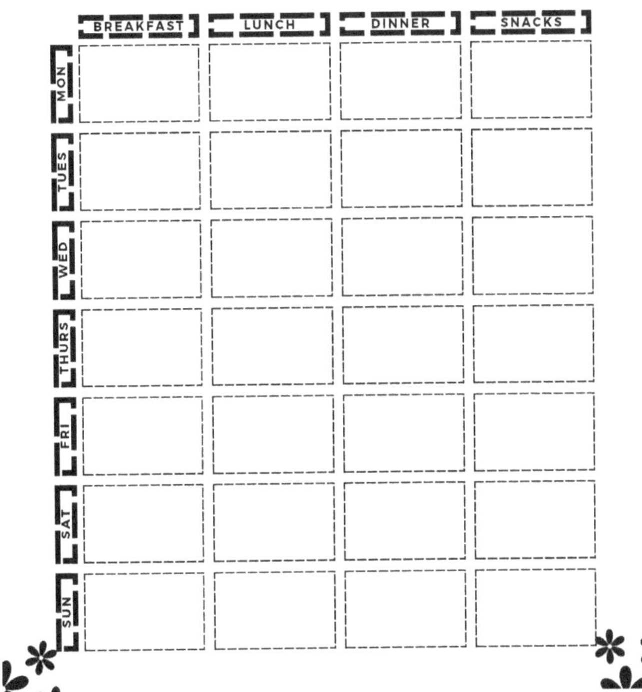

BREAKFAST
LUNCH
DINNER
SNACKS
MON
TUES
WED
THURS
FRI
SAT
SUN

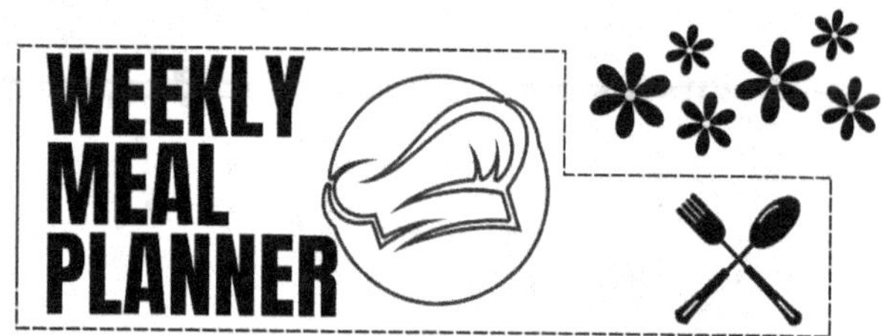

WEEKLY
MEAL
PLANNER

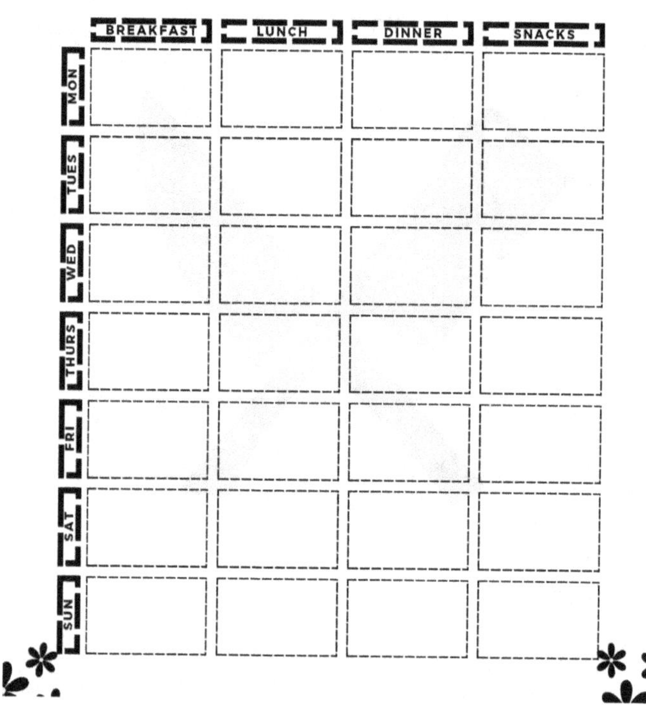

BREAKFAST
LUNCH
DINNER
SNACKS
MON
TUES
WED
THURS
FRI
SAT
SUN